AROMATHERAPY
A Nurses Guide

by Ann Percival

Published by
Amberwood Publishing Ltd
Park Corner, Park Horsley, East Horsley, Surrey KT24 5RZ
Tel: 01483 285919

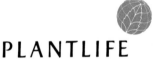

PLANTLIFE

The Natural History Museum, Cromwell Road, London SW7 5BD

Registered Charity No. 328576

Amberwood Publishing supports the Plantlife Charity,
Britain's only charity exclusively dedicated to saving wild plants.

ISBN 1-899308-04-0

Typeset and designed by
Word Perfect, Christchurch, Dorset.

Cover design by Design Hive

Printed in Great Britain

CONTENTS

About the Author

Ann started her training at Paddington General (now St Mary's Hospital) and took up her first staff nurse post at Queen Mary's University Hospital Roehampton.

Firstly on a male surgical ward and then transferring to the Psychiatric Day Hospital. Following the birth of her daughter Francesca she moved with her family to Gloucestershire.

Whilst studying Aromatherapy she worked as a staff nurse, part time, at Cheltenham General Hospital initially on the Cardiology ward and then with the Oncology Unit. She has since presented a series of study days on Aromatherapy for nurses.

She practices from Natural Therapeutics in Cheltenham a specialist shop and clinic run by her husband and runs evening and weekend Introductory Courses on Aromatherapy and Massage.

Acknowledgements

I would like to thank my husband Haydn for his support and encouragement and my daughter Francesca for her interest in aromatherapy and her patience during the time spent writing this book. My thanks to Eve Blundell Consultant Haematologist at Cheltenham General Hospital for her time and help in the writing of the physiology of the immune system. To Maggie Deacon Lead nurse of the Oncology Unit at Cheltenham General Hospital for writing the foreword and for her enthusiasm towards the use of aromatherapy within nursing practice. To a good friend Christabel Burniston for her perceptive proofing and very helpful advice. To the many patients at the hospital that I have nursed and clients at my aromatherapy practice without whom I would not have gained the knowledge to write this book.

Finally to June Crisp for her encouragement.

Note to Reader

Whilst the author has made every effort to ensure that the contents of this book are accurate in every particular, it is not intended to be regarded as a substitute for professional medical advice under treatment. The reader is urged to give careful consideration to any difficulties which he or she is experiencing with their own health and to consult their General Practitioner if uncertain as to its cause or nature. Neither the author nor the publisher can accept any legal responsibility for any health problem which results from use of the self-help methods described.

Foreword

I believe that this book will appeal not only to qualified Aromatherapists and their clients, but also to those with some professional interest in the art of massage and the use of Essential oils. The properties of the various oils are clearly described together with the medical methodology of their safe application.

In my career as a nurse I am particularly aware of the therapeutic value of touch. Unfortunately as medicine becomes more technical we become less tactile with our patients, contact largely being negated by the use of machines. Aromatherapy massage not only provides its own therapeutic benefits through the effects of the oils themselves, but also re-introduces the opportunity for touch which is so necessary for human well-being.

The information contained in this book will enable the reader to increase their knowledge and understanding of the theory, principles and aims of Aromatherapy within the safe, practical and medical context of a 'Nurses Guide'.

Maggie Deacon RGN, Lead Nurse Cancer Centre
Cheltenham General Hospital

1 | Introduction

What is Aromatherapy?

Aromatherapy is the use of pure essential oils which are the life force of the plant. These are extracted from many parts of the plants such as resins, woods, barks, leaves, flowers, berries, cones and the rind of citrus fruits.

Each essential oil has many therapeutic properties which when mixed with a carrier oil is then used for massage to enhance its effects. They can be used in many other ways such as in baths, lotions and vaporisers.

Aromatherapy is an excellent way of maintaining good health, dealing with everyday stress and treating various ailments.

You do not need to be ill to benefit from aromatherapy. Using the oils for home use daily will help to prevent disease, increase mental alertness and maintain your body in equilibrium.

What is Massage?

Massage is the ancient art of touch. It is therapeutic and induces calm, warm, pleasure and relaxation to the mind and the body.

The rhythm of movement over the skin and muscles allows taut, tense muscles to relax and let go.

The movements and depth of the massage can be varied to suit the individual needs.

2 | The use of essential oils

How essential oils work on an emotional level

When essential oils are vaporised we can inhale them because the aromatic molecules are tiny enough to pass directly into the blood stream in the same way as oxygen does. They can have a rapid effect.

The odours stimulate the nerve endings in the Olfactory Bulb which lies at the back of the nose. Here the nerve endings stimulate a part of the brain known as the Limbic System which is in some way associated with our emotions and memories.

The nerve endings in the Limbic system stimulate the Hypothalamus which controls the Pituitary Gland which in turn controls our Endocrine System, responsible for regulating body processes such as reactions to fear, anger, metabolism and sexual stimulus.

By vaporising pure essential oils we can have a positive influence on these reactions by the choice of pure essential oil used.

For example Lavender will calm and help to reduce anxiety whilst Rosemary is a Cephalic stimulant which will promote alertness and aid concentration.

Absorption of essential oils through the skin

For absorption through the skin the pure essential oils must be diluted and mixed with a carrier oil, lotion or cream. Once applied to the skin the aromatic molecules will pass directly through the skin and are absorbed by the body fluids and then circulated around the body in the blood stream.

Some essential oils have an affinity with a particular organ whilst others have a general balancing effect to promote well being of the person. This is determined by the properties of the essential oil used.

The body will use what it needs and then simply excrete the remainder via the lungs and excretory organs.

Carrier oils

These are unperfumed vegetable oils which are cold-pressed and then used as the media to dilute the essential oils for massage use.

Grapeseed Oil is a very commonly used, easily absorbed light carrier oil.

Sweet Almond Oil is extracted from the almond kernel; it is very slightly lighter than grapeseed oil and easily absorbed. It contains vitamins A, B1, B6 and a small amount of vitamin E.

Jojoba Oil is a light golden oil particularly suitable for the face.

Evening Primrose Oil is particularly effective for massage when treating Pre-menstrual Tension, Psoriasis and dry Eczema. Use it as a 25% dilution in conjunction with another carrier oil.

Peach Kernel Oil contains minerals; it is easily absorbed and particularly light for facial use.

Avocado Oil is dark green in colour and is particularly good for dry ageing skin and arthritic conditions. Use as a 25% dilution with another carrier oil.

Wheatgerm Oil is dark orange in colour and rich in vitamin E. It can act as an antioxidant when mixed with other carrier oils and pure essential oil thereby prolonging the life and therapeutic use of the mixed oils. It is particularly good at helping to heal scar tissue.

Essential Oil Notes

Essential oils can be described as either a Top, Middle or a Base Note.

The Top notes are light, stimulating and classed as body energising and uplifting; they also float on top of water.

The Middle notes are levelling, balancing and calming; they are partly soluble in water.

The Base notes are calming, sedative and relaxing; these sink to the bottom in water.

Oils are only 20% soluble in water but are completely soluble in vegetable oil, so once mixed they cannot be separated from the vegetable oil.

To achieve the perfect blend a top, middle and base note oil should be included in your blend.

For example when treating a common ailment such as influenza look at the symptoms:–

Sore Throat. Blocked sinuses.	Eucalyptus top note
Headache. Insomnia.	Lavender middle note
Aching joints.	Benzoin base note

Blending these essential oils with a carrier oil and then massaging into the neck, shoulders, back and aching joints will give considerable relief by helping to stimulate the immune system, relieving the headache, easing the sore throat and aching joints and promoting restful sleep. The synergistic blend of oils works on the whole body to promote recovery.

Ways of using essential oils

There are numerous ways of using essential oils safely and effectively.

Massage – In aromatherapy massage the essential oils are added to a carrier oil such as sweet almond oil before applying to the skin.

Aromatic Baths – These can be relaxing and calming, detoxifying, stimulating and reviving, and give relief to painful muscles.

Fill a bath with water to the temperature you desire then add 6 drops of essential oil. Agitate the water well to disperse the oils then soak for at least 15 minutes.

Footbaths – These are good for athlete's foot or any fungal infection of the feet. Add 3 drops of essential oil to a footbath or a bowl of water then soak the feet for 10 minutes. Always dry the feet thoroughly afterwards.

Sitz Baths – *(or very shallow baths)*. These are ideal for bathing the hips and genital area. Add 4 drops of essential oil and soak for 10 minutes.

Lotions and Creams – These should be pure vegetable based and unperfumed. Any synthetic properties will adulterate and interfere with absorption of the essential oil. Lotions and creams can be made to suit the face and body.

Vaporisation – Vaporisers can be used to vaporise essential oils for inhalation and to deodorise the air. The vapours are simply inhaled just as we inhale oxygen. There are many types of vaporisers available. Each keeps the water hot, with the use of a simple night–light placed in the base of the burner. Add 6 drops of essential oil to the water. The hot water then allows the oils to vaporise the molecules into the air for inhalation.

Steam Inhalation – Essential oils are added to a bowl of steaming hot water; a towel is placed over the head and the vapours are inhaled.

Shampoos – Essential oils can be added to a base unscented shampoo. Once again the shampoo should not have any synthetic detergents in it; the foaming agent is usually coconut palm oil which is a natural foaming agent.

Bubble Bath – The same principle applies here as for shampoos.

Scenting Bed Linen – Add one drop of Lavender to the pillow to aid restful sleep.

Water Sprays – A spray bottle filled with natural spring water can have essential oils added to it, then used as a skin freshener or in a room or a car, as an air freshener.

Compresses – For a hot compress, fill a bowl with 2 pints of very hot water add up to 6 drops of essential oil to it. Immerse a clean flannel into it, wring out and apply it to the area to be treated. Cover it with cling film and a dry towel, leave in place for at least 15 minutes. Remove and very gently massage the area to alleviate any congestion of blood from the site.

To make a cold compress the same principle applies using very cold water.

Diluting and blending essential oils

The recommended concentration is 2½% for adults. Example: 100mls of a carrier oil, lotion or cream; add 50 drops of essential oil to it.

50mls carrier oil; add 25 drops

30mls carrier oil; add 15 drops

20mls carrier oil; add 10 drops

Essential oil bottles always have a "dropper" for easy measuring.

Up to three different essential oils can be blended together.

Children up to eleven years and people with sensitive skin should use a 1¼% dilution

Example: 100mls; add 25 drops

50mls; add 12 drops

30mls; add 7 drops

20mls; add 5 drops

To blend your essential oils with a carrier oil

Fill a dark glass bottle with the amount you need.

Select your essential oils; calculate the number of drops you need to use and add them to the bottle of carrier oil.

Place the lid on it, shake well to blend. Label and date the bottle ready for use.

3 Guide to the definition of the properties of essential oils

Analgesic *Pain Relief:* Lavender, Chamomile (Roman), Rosemary, Ginger.

Anti-Inflammatory *Reduces inflammation:* Chamomile, Lavender, Myrrh, Bergamot.

Antiseptic *Combats bacterial infection locally:* Lavender, Bergamot, Eucalyptus, Tea Tree, Lemon.

Astringent *Tightens the tissues and helps to reduce fluid loss:* Lemon, Cypress, Sandalwood, Myrrh.

Antispasmodic *Helps to reduce muscle spasm:* Chamomile, Lavender, Ginger.

Anti-depressant *Can have an uplifting effect on the nervous system:* Bergamot, Geranium, Orange, Petitgrain

Anti-viral *Will aid in combatting a virus:* Tea Tree.

Bactericidal *Helps to kill bacteria;* Eucalyptus, Lemon, Lavender, Rosemary, Tea Tree, Bergamot.

Bacteriostatic *Helps to inhibit growth of bacteria:* Lavender, Tea Tree, Lemon, Eucalyptus, Bergamot.

Cephalic *Stimulates mental activity:* Peppermint, Rosemary.

Cytophalctic *Aids in cell regeneration:* Lavender, Tea Tree, Neroli.

Carminative *Reduces intestinal spasm:* Ginger, Lavender, Peppermint, Chamomile.

Deodorant *Reduces odour:* Lemongrass, Cypress, Petitgrain, Rosemary.

Detoxifying *Helps to excrete waste products from the body:* Juniper, Lemon, Mandarin.

Decongestant *Relieves congestion:* Eucalyptus, Rosemary, Benzoin.

Emmenagogue *Encourages menstruation (not to be used during pregnancy):* Lavender, Chamomile, Marjoram, Juniper, Clary Sage, Rosemary, Rose, Jasmine.

Expectorant *Helps to expel phlegm:* Eucalyptus, Benzoin, Sandalwood, Bergamot.

Febrifuge *Helps to reduce a fever:* Bergamot, Peppermint, Eucalyptus, Lavender.

Fungicidal *Inhibits the growth of fungi and yeasts:* Tea Tree, Myrrh, Lavender.

Hypertensive *Raises a lowered blood pressure:* Rosemary.

Hypnotic *Helps to induce sleep:* Lavender, Marjoram, Chamomile.

Immuno-stimulant *Helps to strengthen the immune response to infection:* Lavender, Tea Tree, Lemon.

Nervine *Helps to strengthen the nervous system:* Lavender, Rosemary, Marjoram.

Relaxant *Aids mental relaxation:* Chamomile, Clary Sage, Lavender, Marjoram, Ylang Ylang.

Rubefacient *Produces a warming effect when applied to the skin:* Black Pepper, Ginger, Benzoin.

Sedative *Has a calming effect on the nervous system:* Chamomile, Clary Sage, Frankincense, Lavender, Marjoram, Rose.

Stimulant *Has a stimulant effect on the whole body:* Eucalyptus, Geranium, Rosemary, Peppermint.

Uterine *Has a tonic effect on the uterus:* Clary Sage, Rose, Jasmine.

Vasoconstrictor *Causes contraction of capillaries:* Chamomile, Cypress, Lemon, Rose.

Vasodilator *Causes expansion of capillaries:* Marjoram.

Vulinary *Will aid in the healing of wounds:* Benzoin, Bergamot, Lemon, Eucalyptus, Tea Tree, Lavender, Myrrh.

4 | Tables of essential oils

Notes	Therapeutic Properties	Therapeutic Uses	Cautions
Benzoin – Base *Styrax benzoin*	Anti-inflammatory Antiseptic Expectorant Sedative Astringent Vulinary	Skin Care – Cuts, Chapped Skin Poor Circulation Muscles/Joints – Arthritis, Rheumatism Respiratory – Asthma, Bronchitis Coughs, Colds, Sore Throats Immune System – Flu, Colds Nervous System – Stress and Tension	
Bergamot – Top *Citrus bergamia*	Analgesic Antidepressant Antispasmodic Antiseptic Carminative Digestive Laxative Stimulant	Skin Care – Acne, Boils, Cold Sores, Eczema Respiratory – Mouth Infections, Sore Throat Digestive System – Flatulence, Poor Appetite Genito Urinary System – Thrush, Cystitis Immune System – Flu, Colds Nervous System – Depression Anxiety - Stress	Phototoxic. Avoid exposure to direct sunlight
Chamomile Roman – Middle *Anthemis nobilis*	Analgesic Antiseptic Antispasmodic Digestive Febrifuge Nerve Sedative Carminative Bactericidal	Skin Care – Acne, Allergies, Burns, Dermatitis, Eczema, Sensitive Skin, Teething Circulation – Cooling to inflamed joints Muscles/Joints – Arthritis, Rheumatism, Muscular Pain Digestive System – Colic, Indigestion Nervous System – Nervous Tension, Stress, Neuralgia	
Cypress – Middle *Cypressus sempervirens*	Antirheumatic Antiseptic Antispasmodic Astringent Deodorant Diuretic Vasoconstrictive	Skin Care – Oily Skin, Excessive Perspiration Circulation – Varicose Veins, Haemorrhoids, Poor Circulation Nervous System – Nervous Tension, Stress Muscles/Joints – Muscular Cramp, Rheumatism	

Cypress –
Middle
continued

Respiratory System – Asthma, Bronchitis, Spasmodic Coughing Genito Urinary – Painful Periods, Heavy Periods

Eucalyptus globulus – Top

Analgesic
Antineuralgic
Antirheumatic
Antispasmodic
Antiviral
Decongestant
Expectorant
Febrifuge
Rubefacient
Stimulant
Vulnerary

Skin Care – Burns, Blisters, Cold Sores, Skin Infections
Poor Circulation
Muscles/Joints – Rheumatism, Arthritic, Muscular Pain, Sprains
Respiratory System – Coughs, Colds, Sore Throat, Bronchitis, Sinusitis, Catarrh
Immune System – Chicken Pox, Flu, Measles
Nervous System – Neuralgia, Headaches

Frankincense – Base
Boswellia carteri

Anti-inflammatory
Antiseptic
Astringent
Carminative
Digestive
Expectorant
Sedative
Uterine
Vulnerary

Skin Care – Dry Mature Skin, Scars, Wounds
Respiratory – Asthma, Bronchitis, Coughs, Laryngitis
Genito Urinary – Cystitis, Painful Periods
Nervous System – Anxiety
Nervous Tension

Emmenagogue

Geranium – Middle
Pelargonium graveolens

Antidepressant
Anti-inflammatory
Antiseptic
Astringent
Deodorant
Diuretic
Fungicidal
Adrenal Cortex
Stimulant
Vulnerary

Skin Care – Acne, Broken Capillaries, Burns, Dermatitis, Eczema, Ringworm, Wounds
Circulatory – Haemorrhoids, Varicose Veins, Poor Circulation Cellulite
Respiratory System – Sore Throat
Endocrine – Menopause Systems, PMT
Nervous System – Nervous Tension, Neuralgia, Stress

Ginger – Base
Zingiber officinale

Analgesic
Antioxidant
Antiseptic
Antispasmodic
Bactericidal
Carminative
Expectorant
Febrifuge
Laxative
Rubefacient
Stimulant

Poor Circulation
Muscles/Joints – Arthritis, Muscular Aches & Pains, Rheumatism, Sprains Cramp
Respiratory System – Sore Throat, Bronchitis, Sinusitis, Colds
Digestive System – Diarrhoea, Colic Indigestion, Flatulence, Nausea, Cramp
Nervous System – Nervous Exhaustion

Jasmine –
Base
Jasmine officinale

Mild Analgesic
Antidepressant
Anti-inflammatory
Antiseptic
Antispasmodic
Aphrodisiac
Carminative
Sedative
Uterine Tonic

Skin Care – Dry or Greasy Skin,
Sensitive Skin
Respiratory System – Coughs,
Catarrh, Laryngitis
Genito Urinary System – Painful
Periods
Labour Pains – Uterine Disorders
Nervous System – Depression,
Nervous Tension & Stress

Emmenagogue

Juniper –
Middle
Juniperus communis

Antiseptic
Antitoxic
Antispasmodic
Astringent
Carminative
Diuretic
Nervine
Vulnerary
Antirheumatic

Skin Care – Acne, Dermatitis,
Eczema, Wounds, Cellulite
Circulatory – Haemorrhoids,
Arteriosclerosis
Muscles/Joints – Gout,
Rheumatism, Arthritis
Immune System – Flu, Colds,
Infections
Genito Urinary System –
Amenorrhoea, Cystitis,
Dysmenorrhoea
Nervous System – Nervous
Tension & Anxiety

Emmenagogue.
Not to be used
on anyone with
kidney disease

Lavender –
Middle
Lavendula
Augustifolium

Analgesic
Antidepressant
Antirheumatic
Antiseptic
Antispasmodic
Antitoxic
Carminative
Diuretic
Hypotensive
Nervine
Sedative
Vulnerary

Skin Care – Acne, Abscesses,
Allergies, Fungal Infections,
Bruises, Minor Burns, Eczema,
Inflammations, Insect Bites,
Psoriasis, Sunburn, Ringworm
Muscles/Joints – Rheumatism,
Sprains, Aching Muscles
Respiratory System – Asthma,
Bronchitis, Catarrh, Laryngitis,
Throat Infections
Digestive System – Abdominal
Cramps, Colic, Dyspepsia, flatulence
Genito Urinary System – PMT,
Cystitis, Dysmenorrhoea
Immune System – Flu, Colds
Nervous System – Anxiety,
Headache, Insomnia, Migraine

Emmenagogue

Lemon –
Top
Citrus limonum

Antiseptic
Stimulates White
Blood Cells
Antirheumatic
Vermifuge
Antispasmodic
Antitoxic
Astringent
Bactericidal
Carminative

Skin Care – Acne, Boils, Greasy
Skin, Herpes, Insect Bites, Mouth
Ulcers, Warts
Circulatory – Haemorrhoids,
Varicose Veins
Muscles/Joints – Arthritis, High
Blood Pressure, Rheumatism
Respiratory – Asthma, Bronchitis,
Throat Infections
Digestive – Dyspepsia

Phototoxic –
Do not use on
skin exposed to
direct sunlight

16

Lemon –
continued

Diuretic
Haemostatic
Hypotensive

Immune System – Colds, Flu

Mandarin –
Top
Citrus nobilis

Antiseptic
Antispasmodic
Carminative
Digestive &
Lymphatic Tonic
Sedative
Mild Diuretic

Skin Care – Acne, Scars, Spots,
Circulation – Fluid Retention
Digestive System – Dyspepsia,
Hiccoughs
Nervous System – Insomnia
Restlessness, Nervous Tension

Marjoram –
Middle
Origanum
Marjorana

Analgesic
Anaphrodisiac
Antiseptic
Antispasmodic
Antiviral
Bactericidal
Carminative
Digestive
Fungicidal
Hypotensive
Sedative
Vasodilator

Skin Care – Bruises, Chilblains
Circulation – Arteriosclerosis, High
Blood Pressure
Muscles/Joints – Arthritis, Muscular
Aches, Rheumatism, Sprains, Cramp
Respiratory – Bronchitis, Asthma,
Coughs
Digestive – Constipation, Colic,
Flatulence
Genito Urinary – Amenorrhoea,
PMT, Dysmenorrhoea
Immune System – Colds, Flu
Nervous System – Insomnia,
Nervous Tension, Stress

Emmenagogue

Orange –
Top
Citrus aurantium

Antidepressant
Anti-inflammatory
Antiseptic
Bactericidal
Carminative
Digestive
Fungicidal
Digestive & Lymphatic
Stimulant

Skin Care – Mouth Ulcers, Oily
Skin, Cellulite
Respiratory System – Bronchitis
Digestive System – Constipation,
Indigestion, Colic
Immune System – Colds, Flu
Nervous System – Nervous Tension

Phototoxic

Orange
Blossom,
Neroli
Base

Antidepressant
Antiseptic
Antispasmodic
Bactericidal
Carminative
Deodorant
Fungicidal
Mild Hypnotic

Skin Care – Stretch Marks, Scars,
Thread Veins, Sensitive & Mature Skin
Poor Circulation
Digestive System – Diarrhoea,
Flatulence, Colic, Spasms
Nervous System – Anxiety,
Depression, Stress

Peppermint –
Top
Mentha piperita

Analgesic
Anti-inflammatory
Antiseptic
Antispasmodic
Antiviral
Astringent

Skin Care – Acne, Ringworm,
Scabies
Circulatory – Palpitations
Muscles/joints – Muscular Pain
Respiratory System – Asthma,
Bronchitis, Spasmodic Coughs

Emmenagogue

Peppermint –
continued

Carminative
Hepatic
Nervine
Vasoconstrictor

Digestive System – Cramp, Colic,
Indigestion, Flatulence, Nausea
Immune Systems – Colds, Flu
Nervous Tension – Headaches,
Mental Fatigue, Nervous Stress, Vertigo

Black
Pepper –
Middle
Piper nigrum

Analgesic
Antiseptic
Antispasmodic
Antitoxic
Bactericidal
Carminative
Digestive
Diuretic
Rubefacient
Stimulant (Nervous,
Circulatory & Digestive)

Skin Care – Chilblains
Circulatory – Poor Circulation,
Cold Hands/Feet
Muscles/Joints – Rheumatism,
Muscular Aches/Pains, Joint Stiffness,
Sprains, Cramp
Respiratory System – Catarrh
Digestive System – Colic,
Constipation, Flatulence, Diarrhoea
Immune System – Colds, Flu, Viruses

Petitgrain –
Top
Citrus aurantium

Antiseptic
Antispasmodic
Deodorant
Digestive
Nervine
Stimulant

Skin Care – Acne, Excessive
Perspiration, Greasy Skin & Hair
Digestive System – Dyspepsia,
Flatulence
Nervous System – Insomnia
Nervous Exhaustion – Stress

Rose, Damask–
Base
Rosa damascena

Antidepressant
Antiseptic
Antispasmodic
Astringent
Bactericidal
Hepatic Tonic
Uterine Tonic

Skin Care – Broken Veins
(Capillaries), Dry Mature Skin,
Eczema,
Poor Circulation
Respiratory System – Asthma,
Coughs, Hay Fever
Digestive System – Liver
Congestion, Nausea
Genito Urinary System – Irregular
Periods, Uterine Disorders
Nervous System – Depression,
Frigidity, Insomnia, Nervous Tension

Emmenagogue

Rosemary –
Middle
Rosmarinus officinalis

Analgesic
Antirheumatic
Antiseptic
Antispasmodic
Astringent
Carminative
Digestive
Diuretic
Fungicidal
Nervine
Rubefacient
Adrenal Cortex
Stimulant
Tonic to Nervous System
Vulnerary

Skin Care – Acne, Eczema, Greasy
Hair, Stimulates Scalp
Circulation – Arteriosclerosis, Poor
Circulation
Hypotension
Muscles/Joints – Rheumatism
Digestive System – Colitis,
Flatulence, Hepatic Disorders
Genito Urinary – Dysmenorrhoea
Immune System – Colds, Flu
Nervous System – Headaches,
Mental Fatigue,
Nervous Exhaustion, Stress

Emmenagogue
Care with use on
anyone suffering
from high blood
pressure

Sage, Clary –
Top
Salvia sclarea

Anticonvulsive
Antidepressant
Antiseptic
Antispasmodic
Astringent
Carminative
Digestive
Uterine Tonic
Nervine

Skin Care – Acne, Boils, Ulcers
Circulation – High Blood Pressure
Muscles/Joints – Aches & Pains
Respiratory System – Asthma,
Throat Infections
Digestive System – Colic, Flatulence,
Dyspepsia
Genito Urinary – Labour Pains,
Dysmenorrhoea
Nervous System – Depression,
Nervous Tension, Stress

Emmenagogue
Avoid alcohol –
can exaggerate
drunkenness

Sandalwood –
Base
Santalum album

Antidepressant
Antiseptic (Urinary &
Pulmonary)
Antispasmodic
Astringent
Carminative
Diuretic
Sedative
Fungicidal
Tonic (General)

Skin Care – Acne, Dry Skin,
Chapped Skin, Greasy Skin
Respiratory System – Bronchitis,
Catarrh, Coughs, Laryngitis, Sore Throat
Digestive System – Nausea, Diarrhoea
Genito Urinary – Cystitis
Nervous System – Depression,
Insomnia, Stress, Balancing

Tea Tree –
Top
*Melaleuca
alternifolia*

Antiseptic
Antiviral
Bactericidal
Detoxifying
Fungicidal
Immuno-stimulant
Vulnerary

Skin Care – Acne, Abscess,
Athletes Foot, Cold Sores,
Dandruff, Veruccae, Warts,
Wounds
Respiratory System – Asthma,
Bronchitis, Sinusitis
Genito Urinary System – Thrush,
Vaginitis, Cystitis, Pruritis
Immune System – Flu, Colds,
Chicken Pox

Ylang Ylang –
Base
Cananga odorata

Aphrodisiac
Antidepressant
Antiseptic
Nervine
Sedative
Tonic to Circulatory
System

Skin Care – Acne, General Skin
Care
Circulation – High Blood Pressure,
Palpitations
Nervous System – Depression,
Insomnia, Frigidity, Impotence,
Nervous Tension & Stress

5 | The benefits of massage combined with aromatherapy

Massage combined with the use of pure essential oils is an effective way of treating numerous common ailments which can affect different parts of our body. It is also an excellent way of managing stress and for the maintenance of health and general well-being.

You do not have to be ill to benefit from Aromatherapy and Massage. It is a unique and holistic way of promoting and maintaining good health.

The benefits of massage

Revitalised energy

Reduces muscle tension

Stimulates the immune system

Improves the circulation

Improves the circulation of lymph and so helps to excrete waste products

Helps to relieve a headache

Helps to relieve constipation

Helps to prevent cold hands and feet

Helps to prevent cramp attacks

Improves sleep

Gives temporary relief of pain

Helps to reduce stress and anxiety

Aids in relaxation

Assists the response of the body to medical treatment

Promotes a sense of well-being

Massage strokes

Effleurage:

This is a gentle stroking action which has a sedative, calming effect and is particularly good for hyperactivity, nervous and anxious conditions. Effleurage massage helps to lower the blood pressure for short periods.

Light effleurage to the face can alleviate headaches. Firm effleurage is stimulating and helps to improve the blood flow and lymph drainage. The massage brings oxygen to the tissues which improves the nutrients to the area. This is important when treating muscular injuries as contracted muscles have often been affected by a poor blood supply causing a build-up of toxins which need to be cleared.

Technique: Starting on the back, place your hands palm down on the lower back, side by side, gently slide them upwards to the top of the back exerting pressure by leaning on the palms and heels of the hands. When you reach the top of the back fan out at shoulder level and glide down to the base of the back; swivel your hands around and start again.

Petrissage: (Kneading)
Use this technique after the tissues have been warmed up and prepared by effleurage. This movement increases the circulation whilst slightly raising the temperature of the skin thus cleansing the tissues of accumulated waste products.

Technique: Grasp the flesh with one hand and gently squeeze it whilst pushing it towards the other hand. Pick up and squeeze the flesh with the other hand and repeat this sequence round the back or over the thighs.

Wringing:
This helps to separate muscle fibres and release spasms.

Technique: This is similar to kneading but it is deeper and more stimulating. Use the technique for kneading but this time lift the flesh slightly and twist gently.

Taponement:
Stimulating movements such as hacking, cupping, and clapping increase the blood supply locally and raise the skin temperature to the parts being worked on. This helps to break down waste products and is particularly effective for reducing cellulite. (Cellulite is characterised in the puckering of the skin on the outer thighs, hips, and buttocks of females.)

Technique: Hacking – Have the hands outstretched; strike the skin gently but firmly with the sides of your hands alternately. The hands should work quickly; to do this, takes practice to build up the speed.

Cupping – Cup the hands and bring them down one hand after the other in quick movements.

Stroking and rolling:
Gentle relaxing movements.

Technique: With relaxed hands and arms start at the base of the back at the side nearest to you. Begin by pushing inwards with the flat of your hand towards the spine. Work up to the top of the back then lean over and pull the flesh on the other side inwards towards you.

Work across the back at least three times.

Thumb kneading:

The small muscles on either side of the spine can be relaxed by exerting firm but gentle pressure on either side of the spinal column. This will awaken the nerves at either side of the spine and stimulate various organs of the body. Never work directly over the spine.

Technique: Begin at the base of the spine, put your thumb pads either side of the spinal column and work up the back, slowly exerting firm pressure. Release and repeat until you have worked up to the neck; glide down to the base and repeat again.

Circular thumb kneading:

Similar to thumb pressure. You make a circular movement with the thumbs as you work your way up either side of the spinal column.

Giving the massage

Always have warm hands.

Only uncover the part of the body that you are working on.

Try to be as relaxed as possible yourself.

Use the weight of your body to give depth and rhythm to the massage.

Bend your legs when you need to be lower, and not your back.

The masseur should wear loose comfortable clothing for ease of movement.

Keep one hand in contact with the person throughout the massage.

Do not initiate a conversation, leave it to the person who is receiving the massage. Some prefer to enjoy the massage in silence or listening to soft music, whilst others like to chat a little.

Vary the massage stroke from light to firm throughout the massage.

Concentrate on giving the massage and mould your hands to the body, music will help you to pace your rhythm.

Always warm the oils in the palm of your hand before applying to the person's body.

Stiff, lumpy and knotted areas need massage to dispel the tension from the taut tense muscles. Work on them regularly throughout the massage.

The best surface to give a massage on, is a massage couch; if you do not have a couch then a sturdy dining table will do. Check that it will take your weight and that it does not rock. Pad it with blankets so that it is comfortable to lie on.

Remove any jewellery from the person so that it does not impede the free flow of massage movement.

Self-massage

This can be very effective on most parts of the body. It is beneficial to the circulation, flow of lymph and excretion of toxins.

Creating the atmosphere for massage

The room should be warm and well ventilated.

Play some soft gentle relaxing music.

Choose a time when you will not be disturbed.

Vaporise a relaxing essential oil such as Lavender.

Contraindications to massage

Over recent injuries. Ensure that they have been well-healed for a minimum of 12 weeks.

Over tumours or lumps.

Over varicose veins, or phlebitis, or a thrombosis.

Over rheumatic painful joints that are hot to touch and swollen, and never over extensive osteoporosis.

Over skin conditions. Massage can sometimes aggravate the condition.

Over recently fractured limbs or joints.

Immediately before or during a menstrual period. Be careful over the abdomen; massage may increase the flow of blood.

Do not give abdominal massage in cases of diarrhoea, hernia, or colitis. It can aggravate the condition.

If a person has lung disease, use antispasmodic oils.

If a person has haemophilia, massage can cause bruising to the skin.

Percussion movements should not be done over bony areas.

In diabetes, avoid massaging the abdomen.

If a person has a pacemaker avoid the abdomen, neck, and shoulders.

In pregnancy, avoid abdominal massage before the twelfth week of pregnancy. After the twelfth week, choose essential oils that are safe to use during pregnancy. Massage should be given by a qualified aromatherapist.

Cancer

It is quite safe to give a gentle face, hand or foot massage in cancer cases provided there is not a tumour or malignant growth to any of these parts of the body. Larger areas of the body should only be massaged by a qualified aromatherapist and with the consent of both patient and doctor.

How to do a basic back massage

1. Begin at the lower back and gently effleurage 5 times.

2. Knead around the whole back 4 times.

3. Use hacking work around the back 3 times.

4. Follow with cupping work around the back twice.

5. Then stroking and rolling around the back 3 times.

6. Follow with thumb kneading up either side of the spinal column at the lower back. Repeat twice.

7. Proceed with circular thumb kneading up either side of the spinal column once.

8. Move to the top of the person's head and begin effleurage at the shoulders working to the lower back and pull gently upward towards the shoulders. Repeat 3 times.

9. Move to the side of the person and effleurage over the back from the lower back upwards. Repeat 5 times.

10. Finish the massage with gentle stroking movements. Place the palm of the hand downwards at the top of the back of the spinal column, and very gently alternate your hands one after the other, gliding with feather strokes to the base of the back. Repeat 3 times.

11. Now leave the person cosily covered to relax.

How to do a chest massage

Massage can help to relax the chest muscles, relieve muscular tension in the back and shoulders and loosen up the mucous secretions in cases of bronchitis or chesty coughs.

The person should be lying on his/her back.

1. Stand at the head of the person and place your hands on either side of the shoulders and gently press down; this helps to dispel tension.

2. Remain standing at the head of the person and move your hands to the upper centre of the chest, use effleurage stroking downwards to the base of the chest. Swivel your hands in a circular movement around the hips, and pull upwards towards the top of the chest, moving your hands out across the shoulders. Swivel them around to meet in the centre top of the chest and gently glide downwards to the base of the chest area. Repeat 5 times.

3. Stand at the side of the person and effleurage from the centre of the abdomen pushing gently upwards, fanning your hands outwards across the shoulders. Swivel them around and glide down over the chest to the centre. Repeat 4 times.

4. Use stroking and rolling movements from one side of the chest to the other just as you did on the back massage movement No 5.

5. Repeat chest effleurage 5 times as in movement 3.

Now leave the person cosily covered to relax.

How to do a face and neck massage

This massage is good for relieving headaches, improving skin tone and circulation to the face, which is generally an extremely responsive part of the body.

The person can either be lying flat on his or her back or sitting in a comfortable armchair. The therapist should stand at the head of the person.

1. Begin with gentle stroking movements at the base of the neck using the whole palm of your hand and fingers, your hands should be in the prayer position gliding upwards over the chin, across the cheekbones and meeting at the forehead. Repeat 4 times.

2. From the sides of the nose commence gentle stroking movements using the middle and ring fingers of both hands. Work outwards across the cheekbones. Repeat 3 times (this is good for congested sinuses).

3. Stroking from the base of the neck glide upwards over the chin and cheekbones. Pause at the temples, and with gentle circular movements with the tips of the middle and ring finger, gently knead to help to dispel tension. Repeat 5 times.

4. With your knuckles, very gently knead over the cheekbones working outwards.

5. Starting at the chin working with the tips of your middle and ring fingers very gently pat all the way around the outside of the face. This is a stimulating movement. Repeat 3 times.

6. To stimulate the jawline gently pat and slap under the chin with the middle and ring fingers only (this should not be painful).

7. Massage the ears, starting at the lower lobe using the thumb and middle finger. Work around the ear twice.

8. To finish use stroking movements from the base of the neck, gently pulling upwards over the chin, cheekbones and forehead.

Repeat this as many times as you like.

How to do a foot massage

Foot massage can help to relieve tiredness, aching feet, improve the circulation and help to relax the whole body.

1. This massage can be given to the person either on top of a bed, on a couch or sitting in a comfortable armchair. If the person is sitting in an armchair, the therapist should sit down with the person's foot resting on a stool opposite the therapist.

2. Supporting the foot with one hand, apply massage oil to the whole of the foot.

3. Now hold the foot with your left-hand thumb underneath and fingers uppermost. Starting at the base of the large toe gently work your way down the top of the foot between the bones of the foot with circular thumb pressure towards the ankle, glide back to the toes and repeat until you have covered the whole top of the foot.

4. Starting with the big toe, gently rotate it to the right and then to the left. Repeat this to all of the toes.

5. Support the foot with the fingers of both hands, and with the thumbs over the sole of the foot, zig-zag over the base of the foot working from the top of the foot to the heel base.

6. Hold the foot firmly between your hands and begin to stroke the top of the foot with the palms, alternating the hands and massaging towards the body. Repeat 5 times.

7. Hold the foot with the left hand and with the right hand massage the ankle and heel with circular movements. Swap over hands and repeat to the left side of the ankle and heel.

8. Now repeat this massage to the other foot.

How to do an abdominal massage

Abdominal massage should be very gentle to aid relaxation and stimulate a sluggish digestive system.

The person should be lying flat with only the abdomen exposed.

1. Begin with very slow gentle effleurage over the abdomen starting at the lower part with your hands pointing towards the head, gently push upwards over the abdomen, spread your hands out over the top of the abdomen and glide down the sides over the hips bring them down and swivel them around back to the centre of the abdomen. Repeat 3 times.

2. Very gently stroke around the abdomen, palms downwards, in a clockwise direction, (because the intestines move in a clockwise direction), and begin to circle over the abdomen with one hand following the other. Repeat 4 times.

3. Place your hands on the side of the abdomen, opposite to your body, and very gently knead either side of the abdomen. Glide the hands across the abdomen to the opposite side and gently knead this side. Repeat 2 times.

4. With relaxed hands and arms, begin stroking and rolling at the base of the abdomen at the side nearest to you. Begin by pushing gently inwards with the flat of your hand work up to the top of the abdomen. Glide your hands across, and begin by leaning over to the other side of the abdomen and pulling the flesh on the other side towards you. Work over both sides 3 times.

Finish the massage with gentle effleurage 3 times over the abdomen.

6 | Aromatherapy and massage treatments

Muscular and skeletal system

There are two main types of muscles in the body: Voluntary and Involuntary muscles. Voluntary muscles form the flesh of the limbs and trunk and support and move the skeleton. We command these muscles to move.

Involuntary muscles are those which we have no control over. These muscles are controlled by the central nervous system and include those in the walls of the intestines, bladder, bowel and respiratory muscles.

Massage is frequently used to treat many muscular disorders, ranging from muscular aches and pains due to strain, injury or over-use, and degenerative disorders such as osteoarthritis and rheumatism.

Massage can also have an effect on the involuntary muscles due to the reflex effect on the central nervous system. A sluggish digestive system or a raised blood pressure can be helped by massage as a result of its reflex effect on the nervous system.

Conditions frequently helped by massage include back pain due to strain, spasm and stress.

Prevention of aching muscles due to exercise and over-use

Massage of the feet and legs prior to exercise.

Oils to use: Carrier Oil 20 mls
                Add: Rosemary   5 drops
                      Juniper   3 drops
                      Lavender   2 drops.

Pre- and post-exercise lotion

This will help to stimulate the circulation and improve the blood supply to the muscles.

Lotion 100mls Add: Rosemary   25 drops
                     Lavender   12 drops
                     Bergamot   12 drops

Mix well.

Apply before and after exercise to legs, arms and shoulders.

Back pain – Stiff neck and shoulders, also lower back pain due to muscular fatigue, spasm and stress.

MASSAGE TREATMENT: Basic Back Massage
Oils to use:　　 Carrier oil 20 mls
　　　　　　　　 Add: Juniper　　 2 drops
　　　　　　　　　　　 Rosemary　 4 drops
　　　　　　　　　　　 Lavender　　4 drops

Aroma Aids

AROMATIC BATHS using essential oils with calming, analgesic and anti-inflammatory properties such as Lavender, Rosemary, Roman Chamomile and Ginger.

HOT COMPRESSES to the back using oils with the same properties.

BACK PAIN LOTION
100mls lotion　 Add: Bergamot　　 12 drops
　　　　　　　　　　　Rosemary　　25 drops
　　　　　　　　　　　Lavender　　 13 drops

Mix well. Apply to the back, morning and evening, ideally after bathing.

Arthritic joint pains due to wear and tear of the joints, as in Osteoarthritis, can be eased by gentle massage around the painful joints. This will improve the blood supply to the muscles and help to remove any build-up of waste products.

MASSAGE TREATMENT: Gentle stroking and kneading movements around the muscles of the painful joints.
Oils to use:　　 Carrier oil 20 mls
　　　　　　　　 Add: Eucalyptus　 5 drops
　　　　　　　　　　　 Rosemary　　3 drops
　　　　　　　　　　　 Juniper　　　2 drops

Aroma Aids

AROMATIC BATHS using essential oils with warming, analgesic, detoxifying and vasodilatory properties such as Ginger, Rosemary, Marjoram, Lavender and Juniper.

HOT COMPRESSES using the same type of oils.

ANTI-ARTHRITIS LOTION
100mls lotion　 Add: Roman Chamomile　 10 drops
　　　　　　　　　　　Lavender　　　　　25 drops
　　　　　　　　　　　Ginger　　　　　　15 drops

Apply to the aching joints twice daily.

Rheumatoid arthritis often causes inflammation around the joints so massage will be painful. If there is inflammation, and the joints are painful and hot to touch, then massage must not be given.

Compresses and Aromatic Baths using anti-inflammatory and analgesic essential oils have been found by many of my clients to give pain relief. Also use the anti-arthritis lotion 2-3 times a day to help relieve the pain.

Repetitive strain injury

Chronic pain can be caused to the tendons, muscles and joints by overuse, sitting in the same position for long periods and by stress.

MASSAGE TREATMENT
BACK MASSAGE will help to ease the tension in the tight knotted muscles, improve the circulation, bring more nutrients to the painful area and help to excrete waste matter from the muscles.

A gentle hand massage will ease the pain and stiffness and improve the circulation.

Oils to use: Carrier oil 20mls
                 Add: Roman Chamomile   5 drops
                       Lavender   4 drops
                       Juniper   1 drop

Aroma Aids
AROMATIC BATHS: Oils will help the body to unwind and relax, use oils with analgesic and warming properties to relieve pain and improve the circulation: Lavender, Ginger, Benzoin, Juniper and Marjoram.

WARM COMPRESSES will relieve the sore area, using the same type of oils.

LOTION: Once again I can recommend the following lotion to sufferers of Repetitive Strain Injury as it has been found time and time again to help ease discomfort and pain.

Lotion: 100mls Add: Roman Chamomile   15 drops
                      Lavender   17 drops
                      Rosemary   18 drops

Apply the lotion morning and evening to the neck, arms, upper back, shoulders and hands.

Rest the painful joints as much as possible. Walk around for at least 5 minutes in every hour in order to change your body position. Ensure that your seat is comfortable. When you get home after work, take a relaxing bath.

THE DIGESTIVE SYSTEM

The digestive system can be affected by Indigestion, Irritable Bowel Syndrome, Constipation, Bloatedness and a Sluggish Digestive system. All can be helped by Aromatherapy and Massage.

Indigestion is caused when the body does not digest foods adequately and so causes abdominal discomfort. A common cause can be eating too quickly in a stressful environment.

MASSAGE TREATMENT TO RELIEVE AND SOOTHE

Abdominal Massage using slow gentle clockwise strokes around the abdomen.

Oils to use: Carrier Oil 20mls
                  Add: Peppermint 4 drops
                       Lavender 2 drops
                       Ginger 4 drops

Aroma Aids

Vaporise Lavender essential oil to create a calm relaxing atmosphere. If the indigestion is frequent and due to stress, look at the Stress Chapter, and use some of the suggested methods.

Irritable bowel syndrome: Bloatedness, Flatulence and Abdominal Cramps.

MASSAGE TREATMENT: Gentle abdominal massage.

Oils to use: Carrier oil 20mls
                  Add: Peppermint 1 drop
                       Chamomile 4 drops
                       Lavender 5 drops

Aroma Aids

Lotion to relieve bloatedness, flatulence, abdominal cramps and calm and soothe the intestines.

Apply the following lotion to the abdomen morning and night, and massage gently in a clockwise direction.

Lotion: 100mls Add: Lavender 20 drops
                          Peppermint 8 drops
                          Chamomile 12 drops

Constipation and a sluggish digestive system

MASSAGE TREATMENT: An abdominal massage which will stimulate the intestines.

Oils to use: Carrier oil 20mls
                  Add: Lemon 3 drops
                       Rosemary 5 drops
                       Mandarin 2 drops

Aroma Aids
AROMATIC BATHS using stimulating essential oils such as Mandarin, Rosemary and Marjoram.

LOTION FOR CONSTIPATION SUFFERERS
Lotion 100mls Add: Lemon   16 drops
                     Rosemary   15 drops
                     Mandarin   19 drops
This lotion will encourage digestion and relax the intestinal muscles. Drink plenty of fruit juices and mineral water. Ensure that your diet is well-balanced and eat plenty of fresh fruit and vegetables.

Nausea and travel sickness

Preventive Measure: Very gently, massage the abdomen prior to travel, with this blend of oils.
                     Carrier oil 20mls
                Add: Peppermint 5 drops
                     Ginger   5 drops

Aroma Aid
Put a few drops of Peppermint essential oil on a handkerchief and inhale periodically throughout the journey.

CIRCULATORY SYSTEM

The heart pumps blood to all parts of the body via the blood vessels, so providing oxygen and nutrients to all of the organs and body tissues. The circulatory system is also involved in clearing the tissues of waste products.

Massage can improve the circulation by relaxing the tight tense muscles which may be constricting blood vessels thus impairing the flow of nutrients to the organs and muscles. Massage improves the flow of blood, and aids in the cleansing of waste matter from the body organs and tissues. Direct pressure through massage over the blood vessels can aid the return of venous blood to the heart. It can also have a stimulating effect on the nerve endings which control blood vessels.

Conditions that can affect our circulation which can be helped by aromatherapy include: High Blood Pressure, Cramp, Cold hands and feet, Chilblains and Varicose Veins.

High blood pressure or hypertension means that the blood pressure is higher than normal. It occurs when there is resistance in the blood vessels to the flow of blood. If the blood pressure remains consistently raised it will eventually put a strain on the heart; it is therefore regarded as a risk factor for heart disease.

Aromatherapy Massage can lower a raised blood pressure temporarily, especially when the hypertension is caused by stress.

MASSAGE TREATMENT
Use gentle back massage and avoid the stimulating movements of hacking and cupping.

Oils to use: Carrier oil 20mls
                Add: Lavender   5 drops
                       Marjoram   5 drops

Aroma Aids
Vaporise essential oils with calming, sedative properties such as Lavender, Ylang Ylang, Marjoram, and Clary Sage.

AROMATIC BATHS: Use essential oils with relaxant and vaso-dilatory properties such as Lavender and Marjoram to help improve the circulation.

Cold hands and feet can often be due to poor circulation.

MASSAGE TREATMENT
Regular massage of the hands and feet with warming and vaso-dilatory oils will improve the circulation and help to prevent Chilblains from occurring. Massage will also make the stiff hand joints of the elderly more flexible and thus create improved manual dexterity.

Oils to use: Carrier oil 20mls
                Add: Black Pepper   1 drop
                       Marjoram   5 drops
                       Ginger   4 drops

Aroma Aids
AROMATIC BATHS: Use oils with vaso-dilatory and rubeficient properties such as Ginger, Marjoram and Juniper.

FOOTBATHS: Using the same oils.

LOTION: to help improve the circulation:
Lotion 100mls   Add: Black Pepper   5 drops
                       Marjoram   25 drops
                       Ginger   20 drops
Use daily to the hands and feet.

Varicose veins

These are dilated and twisted veins in the legs and are usually a symptom of poor circulation.

MASSAGE TREATMENT

This can improve and strengthen the surrounding veins but *never massage directly over varicose veins*.

It is safe to massage very gently above the affected area of the vein with upward stroking movements. Avoid any stimulating movements. Massage will help to ease aching legs but where varicose veins are present treatment should be administered by a qualified Aromatherapist.

Massage to the feet will help to improve the circulation.

Oils to use: Carrier oil 20mls
             Add: Lemon   2 drops
                    Cypress   3 drops
                    Geranium 5 drops

Aroma Aids

Warm aromatic baths using oils with astringent properties that will help to strengthen the veins. Use Lemon, Camomile or Cypress essential oils.

VARICOSE VEIN LOTION

100mls Lotion Add: Cypress   25 drops
                    Lemon   25 drops

Apply very gently to the affected leg, avoid any pressure over the varicose veins.

Cramp: A cramped muscle is very painful, it is due to the muscle being contracted and impairing the blood flow.

Regular massage of the feet and legs will help to prevent this.

MASSAGE TREATMENT

Foot massage

Oils to use: Carrier oil 20mls
             Add: Black Pepper 1 drop
                    Juniper   4 drops
                    Marjoram   5 drops

Aroma Aids

Aromatic Baths and foot baths with essential oils that have warming, vaso–dilatory and detoxifying properties, will reinforce the massage treatment.

CRAMP LOTION

100mls Lotion Add: Marjoram   25 drops
                    Juniper   13 drops
                    Ginger   12 drops

Apply to the legs and feet daily.

RESPIRATORY SYSTEM

Conditions that can commonly affect the Respiratory System that respond well to aromatherapy are: Coughs, Colds, Sore Throats, Catarrh, Sinusitis and Acute Bronchitis.

Aromatherapy Massage will help to clear and decongest the respiratory tract.

With the use of essential oils that have decongestant, anti-inflammatory, antiseptic, anti-viral and bactericidal properties, the infection will often respond swiftly and positively to the oils while reinforcing the body's natural defence mechanism to combat infection.

MASSAGE TREATMENT

A chest, back and facial massage to aid decongestion, improve circulation, stimulate lymph drainage and bring nutrients to the site of infection.

Oils to use: Carrier oil 20mls
              Add: Eucalyptus 5 drops
                     Tea Tree   3 drops
                     Benzoin   2 drops

Aroma Aids

Vaporise essential oils which have bactericidal, antiseptic and decongestant properties to help break down mucous, decongest blocked sinuses and help to kill airborne bacteria, use oils such as Lemon, Eucalyptus, Tea Tree, Lavender, Rosemary.

STEAM INHALATIONS: To relieve congestion, use Eucalyptus, Rosemary and Tea Tree essential oils.

AROMATIC BATHS: Use essential oils with antiseptic, bactericidal and immuno-stimulant properties such as Rosemary, Tea Tree, Eucalyptus, Lavender and Lemon.

GARGLES: Use 1 drop of Tea Tree oil in a glass of water. Gargle up to 3 times a day. This will combat the infection and help to prevent laryngitis developing.

CHEST RUB: with a lotion.

100mls lotion   Add: Eucalyptus 25 drops
                     Tea Tree   15 drops
                     Benzoin   10 drops

Apply morning and evening before retiring.

THE IMMUNE SYSTEM

The function of the Immune System is to defend against infection. Lower animals have very simple immune mechanisms whereas higher animals have evolved much more sophisticated systems. Humans have flexible and specific methods which provide a more effective response to different infections. The important features are memory, specificity and the recognition of non-self.

The immune system is a complicated network of cell action and reaction throughout the whole body.

The Bone Marrow: This is soft spongy tissue which is found in the bony cavities. Particularly rich sites are the extremities of flat, long and irregular bones (e.g. the pelvis). It contains multi-potent stem cells which can self renew and go on to develop into mature red cells, white cells and platelets.

The Thymus gland: This is a small walnut sized gland which lies behind the breast bone. Stem cells are chemically attracted to the thymus, where they are modified to become T-Lymphocytes (T-cells).

The Spleen: This organ is found in the abdomen lying under the left lower rib cage. It functions as a blood filter removing old worn-out red and white cells. It provides protection against some micro-organisms. It is also a site of antibody production.

The Lymph Nodes: In health these glands or nodes, which occur throughout the body, are very small. During an infection, however, they are enlarged due to increased activity, namely the accumulation of dead white cells and the proliferation of cells actively fighting infection. This is why, for example, the lymph glands around the neck are often found to be enlarged when a throat infection is present.

The Lymphatic system: This is a network which links the organs of the body containing lymphoid tissue, by a series of channels similar to the circulatory system for the blood. It promotes the circulation of lymphocytes and other white cells around the body in the fight against infection.

Cell Types: Macrophages are large blood cells, which are able to ingest bacteria and dead tissue. They are found in the connective tissues and in the walls of the blood vessels, and can roam freely throughout the body helping to keep it clean and free from harmful bacteria. Any organism which is found and cannot be identified will be taken to the T-Memory cells for identification and consequent action.

Lymphocytes: There are two main types: (1) T-Lymphocytes (T-Cells); (2) B-Lymphocytes (B-Cells).

T-Lymphocytes are so-called because they are modified in the thymus. They are responsible for cell-mediated response or cellular immunity.

This means they have the ability to fight infections where the infecting organism has developed the capacity to live and multiply within the cells of the host. (Example as in Tuberculosis)

B-Lymphocytes are so-called because they were originally found to be modified in The Bursa of Fabricus in the chicken. In humans, the modification occurs in the bone marrow.

B-cells and Humoral immunity: The B-cells produce specific antibodies in the lymphoid tissues that circulate in the lymph and blood to reach the site of an attack. If an antibody has already been prepared through a previous invasion on the body then the B-cells can react very quickly by releasing the specific antibody to help bring the invasion swiftly under control. If however, it is a new invader then a new antibody must be made.

When the body is under attack from harmful micro-organisms be it a virus, cancer, or bacteria the immune system will go into action to deal with the invaders.

Conditions that can disrupt the immune system

Stress which is prolonged (or repeated stressors following one another without abatement) and does not allow the body sufficient time to recover and regain its equilibrium can sorely affect the immune system.

Aids: Acquired Immune Deficiency Syndrome because of its destructive effect on the cellular immune system, the sufferer is highly susceptible to infections.

Myalgic Encephalomyelitis (ME)

Immuno-suppressive drugs such as steroids

Anti-cancer Chemotherapy

Long-term use of hormone preparations

Inhalation of tobacco smoke

Exhaust fumes from motor vehicles

Pesticides and drug residues in foods.

Aromatherapy and massage in relation to the immune system

Essential oils can help to strengthen the immune system. There are numerous essential oils which have bactericidal, anti-viral and antiseptic properties which can be vaporised and so inhaled into the circulatory system.

Vaporising essential oils with these properties, will help to kill off some of the airborne bacteria. The essential oils can also be used in lotions, creams and baths, and will then be absorbed through the skin and into the circulatory system.

Oils such as Lavender, Lemon, Tea Tree, Rosemary, Eucalyptus and Sandalwood have a stimulating effect on the immune system.

Lemon helps to activate the white blood cells which are involved in the fight against infections.

Rosemary stimulates the lymphatic system, and has a tonic effect on the circulatory system.

Lavender, Clary Sage, Marjoram and Roman Chamomile all have a sedative and calming effect on the central nervous system and so will induce calm and relaxation which are conducive to healing and repair of body tissues.

The physiological effects of massage on immunity
Massage helps to improve the circulation and stimulates the lymphatic system.

It helps to excrete waste products and toxins from the body.

It promotes good quality sleep.

The psychological effects of massage on immunity
Massage can help to reduce anxiety and tension.

It aids relaxation of both mind and body.

Massage in many cases can improve the response of the body to medical treatment.

COPING WITH STRESS – prevention rather than cure

Regular Aromatherapy Massage using pure essential oils combined with a healthy diet, restful sleep, regular exercise and relaxation will help to maintain your body in a balanced state with an alert refreshed mind and a relaxed body.

Aromatherapy will gently help to maintain the immune system. It will work on the physical and emotional states to maintain health in readiness to recognise and respond swiftly to infections and stress so that disease is kept at bay.

Those of you who are new to Aromatherapy and may already be suffering from some of the manifestations of stress will find that aromatherapy will be able to help alleviate some of the affects.

Common symptoms of stress

Stress can cause muscular aches and pains due to tension and impaired blood flow to the muscles.

The skin can become either dry, or greasy, prone to spots and lacking in tone.

The digestive system can be affected in numerous ways causing a feeling of bloatedness, constipation and generally a sluggish digestive system. This can lead to halitosis (bad breath) and mouth ulcers.

Poor quality sleep can lead to a feeling of irritability, lack of concentration and tiredness.

We can become prone to attacks of infections such as colds, sore throat, and other viral infections because our immune system is weakened.

We feel the need to relax but are unable to 'switch off'. This is usually due to the excessive amount of adrenalin which is pumping around our system.

When we recognise that the body is under stress, and therefore threatened, we can take positive action to alleviate these symptoms. By employing de-stressing techniques to bring our body back into a balanced state conducive to repairing damage, we achieve an alert refreshed mind and a relaxed body.

Aroma Aids

Use the sedative, hypnotic, and anti-depressant essential oils to promote relaxation. These include Lavender, Clary Sage, Roman Chamomile, Orange and Bergamot. These should be used during the evening and other periods of relaxation.

Oils to boost the immune system and therefore strengthen it include Tea Tree, Rosemary, Lemon, Geranium, Eucalyptus.

Vaporise, these oils and use them in Aromatic baths.

Uplifting and stimulating oils to use during the day to aid concentration and promote clarity of thought are:– Peppermint, Rosemary and Lemon.

AROMATIC BATHS

Use stimulating essential oils such as Lemon, Rosemary and Orange during the day and prior to work.

For relaxation and to help unwind, use the calming and sedative oils such as Lavender, Clary Sage, Marjoram and Ylang Ylang.

ANTI-STRESS LOTION to help improve the circulation, ease muscular aches and pains, boost the immune system and for general well being.

100mls Lotion Add: Bergamot   17 drops
                      Lavender   17 drops
                      Rosemary   16 drops

Use this lotion daily, in the morning, particularly on the neck and shoulders.

Skin problems: Facial steaming using bactericidal oils such as Lavender, Bergamot, Geranium and Lemon.

Lotion for the face:–

Lotion 100mls Add: Bergamot   25 drops
                     Lavender   25 drops
The Bergamot is bactericidal and balances the sebum level, and the Lavender is cytophylactic so helps with cell renewal.

Aromatherapy massage treatments

Stimulating back massage for an energising effect.
Use pure essential oils with stimulating properties.
Oils to use: Carrier oil 20mls
                Add: Black Pepper   1 drop
                      Bergamot   4 drops
                      Rosemary   5 drops

A back massage to aid relaxation and promote a good night's sleep
Use oils with sedative, hypnotic and calming properties.
Oils to use: Carrier oil 20mls
                Add: Lavender   5 drops
                      Marjoram or
                      Roman Chamomile   5 drops
Avoid using any stimulating massage techniques.

Abdominal massage for the digestive system to help with bloatedness and indigestion
Use oils with detoxifying and carmative properties such as Mandarin, Juniper, Lavender, Lemon, Peppermint.
Oils to use for a massage:
                Carrier oil 20mls
                Add: Mandarin   3 drops
                      Lavender   4 drops
                      Peppermint 3 drops
Oils for constipation: stimulating and detoxifying oils such as Juniper, Mandarin, Rosemary and Black Pepper.
                Carrier oil 20mls
                Add: Black Pepper   1 drop
                      Juniper   4 drops
                      Rosemary   5 drops

Face massage to help relieve headaches and improve circulation to the face.
                Carrier oil 20mls
                Add: Lavender   5 drops
                      Peppermint 3 drops
It is important to continue to use the essential oils regularly and have massage even when your symptoms have subsided. This will help prevent the symptoms from recurring.

CANCER AND AROMATHERAPY

People who have cancer can often be helped by aromatherapy and massage to ease anxiety and tension, aid relaxation and promote a feeling of general well-being which is all-conducive to healing and coping with the anxiety of the disease.

Anxiety, tension and fear are some of the commonest emotional symptoms which can be persistently with the sufferer. When frightened, we tense our muscles, and in so doing, create pain and shallow breathing; this can then impair the circulation.

Anxiety prevents good quality restful sleep which is necessary for the healing process.

Through massage and the use of essential oils we can help to aid relaxation and deepen and strengthen respiration so improving the circulation. The psychological benefits of aromatherapy will help to ease an anxious mind and uplift a depressed mood. It is important to remember that emotional well-being is as important as the physical health.

Sleep disturbances: People who have cancer can experience difficulty in sleeping well at sometime during their illness. This may be due to emotional anxiety, or to side effects of medication, such as steroids, which can make them become mentally over-active and inhibit sleep. The physical touch of a gentle massage with wonderful smelling oils will help to relax a tense body and an over active mind to give restful sleep. Massage also helps the sufferer to have healing thoughts about his or her body especially when a partner or spouse is the one giving the treatment. This gentle non-invasive physical contact is soothing to both mind and body. It is a positive way a partner can feel involved in the care of a loved one.

Vaporise essential oils in the bedroom that have a calming and sedative effect on the central nervous system, such as Lavender and Ylang Ylang.

Provided the person's doctor has no objection, then an Aromatherapist can give gentle massage and also show a relative some simple massage techniques.

This massage treatment could be a hand, foot, back or face massage.

Oils to use: Carrier oil 20mls
                 Add: Lavender   5 drops
                       Mandarin   2 drops

It is important that massage is not performed by an untrained person on any part of the body that is swollen or oedematous.

Sore mouth: Mouth ulcers can occur in people who are receiving chemotherapy. It is better to try and prevent ulcers forming by keeping the mouth and gums as clean as possible. After eating rinse the mouth with a Tea Tree mouth wash.

To make this, fill a tumbler with water. Add 1 drop of Tea Tree pure essential oil mix well. Rinse the mouth thoroughly holding the mixture/mouthwash in the mouth for a few seconds at a time.

Drink plenty of fresh fruit juices and mineral water throughout the day. Sometimes antibiotics are prescribed for infections, and they can occasionally cause a fungal infection called Thrush to develop in the mouth making it very unpleasant and sore. The Tea Tree mouth wash in conjunction with any medication the doctor may prescribe will help to combat this.

Constipation: To prevent this, the patient should eat a well-balanced diet and drink plenty of fluids. Very gentle abdominal massage can sometimes be of help to promote peristalsis. Should the patient experience any pain or discomfort from the massage then the massage should be stopped immediately.

Chemotherapy: Chemotherapy for cancer is treatment with cytotoxic drugs. It can have an adverse effect on the white blood cells which help to protect the body from bacteria by fighting infection. This can result in the person being more susceptible to contracting colds, sore throats and other infections, particularly when in close contact with other people. Crowds should be avoided.

Vaporising essential oils at home that have bactericidal and antiseptic properties such as Eucalyptus, Lemon, Tea Tree and Lavender will give the body some protection against airborne bacteria. These oils could also be vaporised in a working environment.

When attending for chemotherapy at the hospital shake a few drops of Lavender essential oil onto a handkerchief and then inhale it periodically whilst waiting to receive treatment. The Lavender oil will have a calming effect on the nervous system and will also act as a respiratory antiseptic.

Vaporising essential oils that have calming and relaxing properties on the emotions used prior to going for the chemotherapy treatment will help to reduce anxiety and calm an anxious mind.

Receiving chemotherapy is a stressful and tiring experience for most people. Therefore, an aromatherapy massage preceding or following the treatment can help to ease tension and aid relaxation. This need only be a gentle massage to the face, back or feet to have a beneficial effect.

Skin problems: Itchy or dry skin can be due to the cancer or sometimes the treatment. Either way, it is another problem which can prevent sleep and rest. The use of a pure vegetable-based lotion with an anti-inflammatory essential oil added to it can often soothe an inflamed and irritated skin. The lotion I would suggest is 100mls Base Lotion plus a 1% dilution of Roman Chamomile added to it. Before applying to a large part of the skin, try a patch test and leave for two hours. If there is not adverse skin reaction then apply the lotion to the irritated skin.

To make: 100mls of pure unscented base vegetable lotion add 20 drops of Roman Chamomile essential oil and shake well.

Respiratory problems: Shortness of breath and coughing can be due to the illness especially in the case of lung cancer. To complement treatment given by the doctor, vaporising essential oils that have decongestant and mucolyptic properties, will help to relieve congestion caused by thick mucous. Oils to use are Eucalyptus, Rosemary and Benzoin.

Aroma aids to help with emotional well-being

Vaporise essential oils which have uplifting, antidepressant, calming and relaxing properties.

Oils to use: Lavender, Orange, Mandarin, Bergamot, Geranium, Lemon, Grapefruit.

Vaporise essential oils to help with sleep such as Lavender, Marjoram.

Put a drop of Lavender essential oil on the pillow at night. Inhaling the essential oil vapour that is on the pillow will aid relaxation.

AROMATIC BATHS

If bathing is allowed and the person is physically able to bathe, then this will promote restful sleep. Oils to use are Lavender, Clary Sage, Ylang Ylang or Chamomile Roman. Fill the bath with water to an agreeable temperature; then, add 6 drops of essential oil and relax in the bath for at least 15 minutes.

Patients in hospital who are unable to take a bath due to the effects of the illness can still enjoy the benefits of essential oils. The nurse can add 2 drops of Lavender or Mandarin essential oil to the bowl of water she will use to give the patient a blanket bath.

Carers need care too

Once again we should not forget the carers who can get very tired and in need of an emotional lift, so a professional Aromatherapy massage once a month will give a physical and emotional boost.

CORONARY ARTERY DISEASE AND HEART ATTACK

Arteriosclerosis is caused by a slow build-up of fatty deposits in the lining of the coronary arteries leading to the heart. It causes narrowing in parts of the arteries and can impede the normal flow of blood and oxygen to the heart. This can lead to a condition known as Angina, a pain in the chest brought on usually following exercise and sometimes stress.

Because blood flow is slowed down due to the narrowing of the arteries, a clot may form on the inner roughened walls of any of the coronary arteries resulting in blocking the supply of blood and oxygen to some of the heart muscle. This causes excruciating pain in the chest, other symptoms may be nausea and a fall in the blood pressure and is known as a heart attack. This is always treated as an emergency.

Following the attack the victim is frequently frightened, exhausted and anxious. Medical treatment should be given immediately to alleviate this. After the acute phase is over and the patient is responding well to treatment, it is the anxiety that usually resurfaces. Some patients are more fortunate, and following investigations, it is found that they have not suffered a heart attack, they have experienced severe chest pains but there has not been a myocardial infarction which causes a part of the heart muscle to die. The person has received a warning that they need to slow down and re-evaluate their lifestyle.

Aromatherapy can be a valuable therapy to incorporate into the lifestyle to help potential heart patients.

Before the patient goes home, a nurse will spend some time discussing, amongst other things, the importance of relaxation and managing their lifestyle in order to prevent the possibility of a further attack in the future. The nurse will help the patient to identify things which are found to be particularly stressful; to plan the day in such a way that time is managed better, alleviating the need to rush around. Patients should practise relaxation by taking a relaxing bath at the end of each day, using essential oils such as Lavender, Marjoram, or Ylang Ylang in the bath. All of these oils have a calming effect on the central nervous system and so will help to aid relaxation. This bath should be taken at a time when other family members will not interrupt. Play some favourite relaxing music; put candles in the bathroom to give a subdued effect and vaporise a relaxing essential oil. Enjoy the bath for at least half an hour. This will help to wind down a tired body and create a wonderful relaxing effect on all the senses. It should become a daily habit.

Whilst the patient is in hospital, the nurse or a relative could give a gentle hand massage. I have found that this often leads the patient to express anxieties which they have been suppressing. These anxieties frequently can be resolved, thus allowing the patient to feel in a calmer state which is conducive to a good recovery.

For a hand massage:

             Carrier oil 10mls
             Add: Lavender   5 drops

Sometimes medication to help with sleep can be avoided or reduced. Many patients have found that a drop of Lavender oil on the pillow helps to promote a good night's sleep. This can then be practised when the patient goes home.

Use Essential oils, at home during the day, that are energising and uplifting such as Orange, Bergamot and Lemon. During the evening switch to the oils that have relaxant properties such as Lavender and Cedarwood.

Massage is therapeutic in many ways. A gentle back massage could be given by the patient's partner on return to their home. Alternatively, the person could visit a professional aromatherapist for a massage. Many people find that having a massage once a month can have a profound effect on their general well being.

BACK MASSAGE

Oils to use: Carrier oil 20mls
               Add: Lavender   10 drops

Often, the relatives are tired and feeling the strain following the experience of a loved one having a heart attack. They, too, would benefit immensely from a massage and the use of essential oils to boost their confidence and promote general well-being. Aromatherapy combined with gentle exercise, a healthy diet and relaxation will aid recovery and help to ensure future good health.

7 | Index of physical conditions

Methods of Use: M-Massage B-Bath I-Inhalation G-Gargle C-Compress V-Vaporise

Digestive System	*Method of use*	*Essential Oils*
Bloatedness	B M C	Peppermint, Mandarin, Ginger
Constipation	M B C	Mandarin, Rosemary, Black Pepper
Diarrhoea	B C	Chamomile, Lavender
Indigestion	B M C	Peppermint, Rosemary, Lavender
Mouth Ulcers	G	Tea Tree
Oral Thrush	G	Tea Tree

Circulatory System		
Colds hands & Feet	M B	Ginger, Marjoram, Black Pepper
Varicose Veins	B C	Lemon, Cypress
Hypertension	M B	Lavender, Marjoram
Cramp	M B	Ginger, Chamomile, Lavender, Juniper
Palpitations	M B	Ylang Ylang, Lavender

Respiratory System		
Coughs	M B I V	Eucalyptus, Sandalwood, Benzoin
Asthma	M B	
Sore Throat	M B I V	Tea Tree, Eucalyptus, Benzoin
Sinusitis	M B I V	Eucalyptus, Rosemary, Lemon, Tea Tree
Acute Bronchitis	M B I V	Benzoin, Sandalwood, Eucalyptus

·Muscular/Skeletal System		
Pre-exercise	M B	Lavender, Bergamot, Rosemary
Post-exercise	M B	Bergamot, Lavender, Marjoram
Muscular Strain	M B C	Lavender, Black Pepper, Bergamot, Rosemary
Backache	M B C	Juniper, Lavender, Rosemary
Rheumatoid Arthritis	B C	Juniper, Chamomile, Lavender
Osteo-arthritis	M B C	Lavender, Black Pepper, Juniper
Repetitive Strain Injury	M B C	Rosemary, Chamomile, Bergamot

Immune System		
Colds	M B I V	Eucalyptus, Lavender, Rosemary
Influenza	M B I	Tea Tree, Benzoin, Lavender
Boosting Immunity	M B I	Tea Tree, Lemon, Eucalyptus, Lavender

OTHER BOOKS FROM AMBERWOOD PUBLISHING ARE:

Aromatherapy – A Guide for Home Use by Christine Westwood. All you need to know about essential oils and using them. £1.99.

Aromatherapy – For Stress Management by Christine Westwood. Covering the use of essential oils for everyday stress-related problems. £2.99.

Aromatherapy – For Healthy Legs and Feet by Christine Westwood. A comprehensive guide to the use of essential oils for the treatment of legs and feet, including illustrated massage instructions. £2.99.

Aromatherapy – Simply For You by Marion Del Gaudio Mak. A clear, simple and comprehensive guide to Aromatherapy for beginners. £1.99.

Aromatherapy – A Nurses Guide for Women by Ann Percival SRN. Building on the success of her first 'Nurses Guide', this book concentrates on women's health for all ages. Including sections on PMT, menopause, infertility, cellulite. Everything a woman needs to know about healthcare using aromatherapy. £2.99.

Aroma Science – The Chemistry & Bioactivity of Essential Oils by Dr Maria Lis-Balchin. With a comprehensive list of the Oils and scientific analysis – a must for all with an interest in the science of Aromatherapy. Includes sections on methodology, the sense of smell and the history of Aromatherapy. £4.99.

Plant Medicine – A Guide for Home Use (New Edition) by Charlotte Mitchell MNIMH. A guide to home use giving an insight into the wonderful healing qualities of plants. £2.99.

Woman Medicine – Vitex Agnus Castus by Simon Mills MA, FNIMH. The wonderful story of the herb that has been used for centuries in the treatment of women's problems. £2.99.

Ancient Medicine – Ginkgo Biloba (New Edition) by Dr Desmond Corrigan BSc(Pharms), MA, Phd, FLS, FPSI. Improved memory, circulation and concentration are associated in this book with medicine from this fascinating tree. £2.99.

Indian Medicine – The Immune System by Dr Desmond Corrigan BSc(Pharms), MA, Phd, FLS, FPSI. An intriguing account of the history and science of the plant called Echinacea and its power to influence the immune system. £2.99.

Herbal Medicine for Sleep & Relaxation by Dr Desmond Corrigan BSc(Pharms), MA, PhD, FLS, FPSI. An expertly written guide to the natural sedatives as an alternative to orthodox drug therapies, drawing on the latest medical research, presented in an easy reference format. £2.99.

Herbal First Aid by Andrew Chevallier BA, MNIMH. A beautifully clear reference book of natural remedies and general first aid in the home. £2.99.

Natural Taste – Herbal Teas, A Guide for Home Use by Andrew Chevallier BA, MNIMH. This charmingly illustrated book contains a comprehensive compendium of Herbal Teas gives information on how to make it, its benefits, history and folklore. £2.99.

Garlic– How Garlic Protects Your Heart by Prof E. Ernst MD, PhD. Used as a medicine for over 4500 years, this book examines the latest scientific evidence supporting Garlic's effect in reducing cardiovascular disease, the Western World's number one killer. £3.99.

Insomnia – Doctor I Can't Sleep by Dr Adrian Williams FRCP. Written by one of the world's leading sleep experts, Dr Williams explains the phenomenon of sleep and sleeping disorders and gives advice on treatment. With 25% of the adult population reporting difficulties sleeping – this book will be essential reading for many. £2.99.

Signs & Symptoms of Vitamin Deficiency by Dr Leonard Mervyn BSc, PhD, C.Chem, FRCS. A home guide for self diagnosis which explains and assesses Vitamin Therapy for the prevention of a wide variety of diseases and illnesses. £2.99.

Causes & Prevention of Vitamin Deficiency by Dr Leonard Mervyn BSc, PhD, C.Chem, FRCS. A home guide to the Vitamin content of foods and the depletion caused by cooking, storage and processing. It includes advice for those whose needs are increased due to lifestyle, illness etc. £2.99.

Eyecare Eyewear – For Better Vision by Mark Rossi Bsc, MBCO. A complete guide to eyecare and eyewear including an assessment of the types of spectacles and contact lenses available and the latest corrective surgical procedures. £3.99.